Dedication

This book is dedicated to my family first. Robert, my love, you've taught me more about love, life, loyalty, and dedication than I ever imagined. Gabriel, Matthew, and Marie Clare, my other loves, may you continue to blossom into the amazing beings you were created to be without apology for being who you are.

This is also dedicated to the thousands of clients I've had the privilege to be of service to. You are some of the bravest, most courageous people I've ever met.

*And, of course, I dedicate this to you, the reader, for investing in yourself, for taking the time to read this valuable resource to find **your** voice and free the immense power that lies within you.*

Stop by our Itty Bitty™ website to find interesting information regarding Finding Your Voice at:

www.IttyBittyPublishing.com

Or visit Sloane Reali at

www.VocalCoachingBySloane.com

Your Amazing
Itty Bitty™
Find Your Voice
and
Transform Your
Life

15 Ways to Instantly Access the
Power of Your Voice

Sloane Reali

Published by Itty Bitty™ Publishing
A subsidiary of S & P Productions, Inc.

Printed in the United States of America

Itty Bitty Publishing
311 Main Street, Suite D
El Segundo, CA 90245
(310) 640-8885

ISBN: 978-1-959964-90-2

Disclaimer: Voice exercises should be done in
five-to-ten-minute increments or less and spaced
throughout the day. If your voice tires or your
throat feels rough or scratchy, you are probably
overdoing the exercises or doing them incorrectly. Vocal Coaching by Sloane or the publisher
does not assume any responsibility for injury to a
reader's vocal apparatus that results from overdoing or incorrectly performing the exercises
described in this book.

Table of Contents

Introduction

Exercise 1.   Find Your Voice, Free Your Power

Exercise 2.   I Feel Naked and Out of Control

Exercise 3.   What Julia Child, Nat King Cole, and Alicia Keys Have in Common

Exercise 4.   Try This if You Frequently Need to Repeat Yourself

Exercise 5.   Just Breathe: Everything You Need to Know About Breathing

Exercise 6.   Vibrato: Your Voice Wants to Support You

Exercise 7.   Never Lose Your Voice Again!

Exercise 8.   Pitch: Are You Monotonous or Melodious?

Exercise 9.   The Five Elements: What Does Your Voice Say About You?

Exercise 10.   Seven Chakras to Reduce Stress, Improve Your Health, and So Much More

Exercise 11.   Recording: Be the Star You Already Are!

Exercise 12.   Listening: You Have Two Ears and One Mouth; Use Them in Proportion

Exercise 13.   Performing/Presenting: Conquer Fear for Good

Exercise 14.   The Gift of Meditation and Movement

Exercise 15.   Pick Up the Mic and Get on the Stage!

Introduction

The book you hold in your hands is a mere glimpse of over two decades of work with thousands of courageous people just like you. They reached out because they were suffering from vocal health issues. They came because they had enough of being passed over for the next promotion or not getting the raise they had planned for. They called because they were sick of being treated like a doormat in their relationships (needing to stand up for themselves) and believed deep down there was something better.

If you can relate to any of the above, this book is your jumping-off point. It is a tool to catapult you into the life you've always desired. Whether you're a singer wanting to bring your best performance to the stage or a business owner desiring to motivate your company's management and employees to buy into bigger picture goals for the company, the methods taught in this book will change the trajectory and transform your life if you practice them consistently.

Exercise #1
Find Your Voice, Free Your Power

The number one fear today continues to be public speaking, let alone singing. With an estimated seven seconds to connect with your listener on any level, by using even a handful of the exercises here, you have the power to inspire, motivate, or challenge any audience of any size to take action and effect change on a massive scale.

1. You essentially have **one voice** you can access from different places in your body by using your breath and energy.
2. Throw in some focused mindful attention and the results are instant and amazing.
3. Anything you do with your voice requires air moving through the vocal cords to make them vibrate and create the sound that is your voice.
4. Using your voice is a physical, mental, sometimes very personal, and even spiritual act.
5. It is helpful to know where and when you don't fully show up or use your voice to get the best results. By doing the exercises here you will be able to access your best voice even in times of stress.

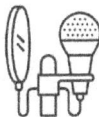

More About How to Find Your Voice

You're in the right place if:

- You have difficulty speaking or communicating your ideas.
- You've been told to, "Speak up, I can't hear you," and felt embarrassed because you **know** you have valuable contributions to make; you just can't get them out.
- Words literally get stuck in your throat.
- At the end of the day, your throat is sore, tired, or fatigued.
- You've always wanted to learn to sing but were told you're tone-deaf. Ouch!
- You're afraid of being judged when speaking up, singing in front of others, showing up, and being who you truly are.
- You've tried vocal work on your own using YouTube, TikTok, etc., and maybe had some success, but it didn't last.

Exercise #2
I Feel Naked and Out of Control

The first body area we will explore is what I refer to as your **low-voice.** This is the first of what I call your three vocal vicinities. They sit in the lower region of your body from your rib cage down, comprised of your first chakra (base), second chakra (sacral), and third chakra (solar plexus).

1. For this exercise, place your hands on your abdomen at or below your belly button. Take a deep breath, filling your solar plexus muscle, causing your hands to rise on the inhale and lower on the exhale. NOTE: This prevents shallow breathing, which is the raising of your chest and shoulders to your ears.
2. Next, exhale with your mouth closed and hum to create vibration with your vocal cords into the lowest part of your body. Relax as you breathe in through the mouth while exhaling through the nose, humming simultaneously. See how low you can go.

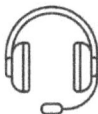

More About Your Low Voice

The ability to relax is a significant key to accessing your full voice. The more relaxed you are the lower you'll be able to go. Keep this in mind as you continue reading and applying these principles to your voice until you feel you've reached the absolute bottom or lowest register of your low voice.

Other ways to access your low voice:

- Visualize your breath as stair steps or imagine taking an elevator down to the basement of your belly.
- Say affirmations such as, "I am connected with energy and supported by Mother Earth."
- Try yawning starting at the top of your head and relaxing all the way down to the bottoms of your feet.

Exercise #3
What Julia Child, Nat King Cole, and Alicia Keys Have in Common

Next up is your **mid-voice,** also known as your speaking voice. Depending on the activity you're doing, for singers this voice can be used to belt out big dramatic songs. You can cheer for your favorite team at an athletic event, or inspire a group or audience as a motivational speaker.

1. To access this part of your voice, begin with the deep breath you used in Exercise #2, filling your solar plexus as you draw your breath down while expanding your belly out and forward.
2. On the exhale, open your mouth, drop your jaw, and create the sound "ahh" from your chest area. Continue using your breath and energy to create volume and sound. **Important:** If you're not used to "getting loud," this is a great way to practice moving through your beliefs relative to your voice.
3. Continue this for a dozen repetitions, inhaling down and out, then exhaling loudly from your chest area with the sound "ahh."

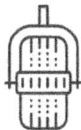

More About Finding Your Mid-Voice

Here are a few things to consider in accessing this part of your voice.

- Allow yourself to get loud!
- You'll likely feel a bit silly and self-conscious. This is all part of the break-through on this journey.
- At this point, everything is about moving big energy out of your body, as opposed to sounding a particular way.
- Try to have fun with this as you explore and experience your voice in a new manner.
- In fact, the feedback I often receive when doing this exercise with clients is that it "feels good, like a giant release of built-up tension in their body."
- Remember to have fun with these exercises and that it's okay to laugh if you feel moved to do so.
- Finally, try not to take all of this so seriously and enjoy the ride.

Exercise #4
Try This if You Frequently Need to Repeat Yourself

Your **high-voice** is in your head. Unlike voices in your head, but rather your high voice, also known as the falsetto.

1. To reach this part of your voice—you guessed it—start with that deep belly breath inhaling down and out into your solar plexus.
2. Next, draw on the breath like a giant straw running through your body, and on the exhale, create the sound "whooo" and gently release the sound like a siren from the top of your head. **Note:** If you do this with too much energy, the extra energy will keep you in your chest voice. Stay relaxed and don't worry about your vocal break or voice cracking. More on that later.

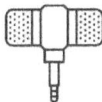

More About Your High Voice

- The key is to come from a place of relaxation. You never want to push or force anything to happen with your voice.
- Pro tip: *Forcing* your voice to do anything could potentially cause several problems, as is the case if you've been to a rock concert or event where you tried to communicate over the level of sound and found yourself hoarse the next day.
- Continue in this pattern for 10-12 repetitions, each time trying to get a little higher than before. Have fun, be playful, and try not to worry too much about the sounds you're creating. At this point, you are just moving energy around in your body using your voice.

Exercise #5
Just Breathe:
Everything You Need to Know About Breathing

Most people on the planet are disconnected from their diaphragm. Instead, their breath is shallow, and they often hyperventilate, or even worse, hold their breath. I teach a four-point technique that guarantees immediate measurable results when adhered to. These are some of the tools in your voice toolbox. I refer to them as the four Ps, known as 1) pant breath, 2) body pulsing, 3) open forward placement, (aka projection,) and 4) pitch. Let's begin with **pant breath**.

1. Breath is life. Without oxygen, a human being cannot live. Did you know brain damage starts within two minutes, and you're dead within five? Not just breathing, but breathing correctly is vital to your very being.
2. Let's go back to Exercise #2. For this exercise, place your hands on your abdomen at or below your navel.
3. Next, take a deep breath filling your solar plexus and causing your hands to rise on the inhale and lower toward your spine on the exhale.

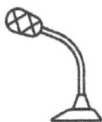

More About Correct Breathing

If this is still challenging, try lying on the floor, and placing a large book or binder on your stomach. Your goal is to make the binder rise toward the ceiling on your inhale and lower to the floor on your exhale. Please be patient with yourself if this takes a few minutes to figure out. You will get it. I've had 100 percent success with this exercise, every single time!

- Now let's do some pant breathing. Either lie on the floor with a binder on your belly or stand with your hands on your solar plexus.
- The sensation at your throat should be that of "ha, ha, ha, ha, haaa" as you exhale five times releasing the last bit of air from your solar plexus.
- Continue this pattern 10-20 times. As you get more comfortable building strength and endurance as you go, you'll be able to increase speed and do more repetitions.

Please note, never sacrifice proper technique by going faster. This will turn little things into bigger problems later. Take your time. Have fun with this.

Exercise #6
Vibrato:
Your Voice Wants to Support You

The second tool in your toolbox is **body pulsing**. Simply put, this is the human body's natural propulsion system for moving air through your vocal cords to make them vibrate and produce sound. For singers, using the vibrato allows them to hold long notes even longer.

1. To access your vibrato, you will continue to draw breath down and forward into your solar plexus on the inhale.
2. Let's add another piece that helps connect your "mental brain" to your physical body with what I call a power punch. Using your dominant hand, throw a punch forward, attaching the "ah" sound at full extension of your arm five times. "Ah, ah, ah, ah, ah", on the exhale.
3. Repeat this pattern 10-12 times. Take a deep breath in between each run as you continue to simultaneously throw your punch along with your voice, "ah," releasing everything at the end of the fifth repetition.

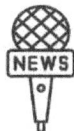

More About Body Pulsing and Vibrato

You literally slow down your body's natural mechanism so you're in control instead of on auto pilot. You always draw air and energy from your solar plexus to produce sound, not from your chest and never from your throat.

Although the use of vibrato is primarily for singers, I include it here as a vocal exercise and another way of connecting with your voice. If you're a singer, having access to and using this tool correctly is critical to avoiding vocal strain. It's the difference between pulling a chord or rope tightly versus loose and relaxed like a wave of sound.

Keys to using your vibrato safely and correctly:

- Practice good breath control originating from your solar plexus, never from your throat.
- Use your vibrato sparingly. A little goes a long way.
- Stay relaxed; never push or force. Pushing or forcing will only result in tension and strain.
- Have fun, play with this, and try not to pass judgment. It's a journey.

Exercise #7
Never Lose Your Voice Again!

Open forward placement (projection) is the second most important tool in your vocal toolbox. It's the difference between what it feels and sounds like in your throat when you make the short vowel sound "a" in words like "at, that, cat." However, this is not the sound we're going for, but rather the opposite sound of "awe" you make with words like "awesome, audible, or audacious."

1. To begin, stand in front of a mirror so you can see the shape you create using your jaw, lips, teeth, and tongue.
2. Next, drop your jaw open, and move your jaw slightly forward, creating a horn shape with your lips.
3. Lastly, play with different shapes to create different sounds. In this case, use the vowels in the English language A, E, I, O and U.

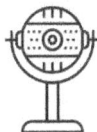

More About Never Losing Your Voice Again

- Now let's play. First, draw your breath down and out into your solar plexus. (Remember the binder?)
- As you exhale, imagine you're a giant oak tree, and instead of drawing water and nutrients from the soil, draw air and energy from the bottoms of your feet up through your legs, your solar plexus, lungs, and then release the long A sound (as in ape) to create an open and forward-placed or projected vowel A.
- Repeat this process for the rest of the vowels: equal for E, idle for I, and open for O. You get the idea.

This step combined with correct breathing is a game changer. If this is the only piece you incorporate with this new knowledge, it will correct and prevent a multitude of vocal challenges, including but not limited to vocal fatigue, vocal fry, losing your voice, and VCD (vocal cord dysfunction), to name a few.

Exercise #8
Pitch:
Are You Monotonous or Melodious?

Everything is vibration—you, me, the chair you are sitting on, the sounds you hear. Frequency is the scientific term for what we refer to as pitch in music or the spoken word as perceived by your ears. For singing, **pitch** is about being able to hear a note and finding it. Pitch for speaking is a little different in that it's more connected to tone and timing. We will address both in this section.

1. Pitch for singing is a matter of one of two things. 1) You need to relax, which is the case if you give more energy than needed, causing you to overshoot the desired note, making it sharp (#). 2) You need to produce more air, energy, and athleticism to prevent falling flat (b), not allowing yourself to reach the note.

2. Pitch for speaking is a matter of how slow or fast you speak. Do you speak at the same volume in the same tone, at a mumble, or at a low droning pace that puts people to sleep? Would you like to be able to share stories or jokes that elicit interest and curiosity from others?

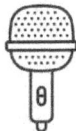

More About Pitch

When you're nervous or anxious, do you speak in a higher-pitched tone causing you to lack authority? For example, does this happen when you make presentations or lead meetings?

- The remedy? You guessed it. Take five to ten deep breaths into your solar plexus to find your center and begin from a relaxed place, instead of from a place of tension.
- The solar plexus is located above your navel and below your rib cage.
- When taking your deep breaths avoid raising your shoulders to your ears and instead draw the breath down and out, expanding your belly forward.
- This is how to correctly engage the solar plexus.
- We will do more with this in the next chapter on the five elements where we will play with different character voices.

Exercise #9
The Five Elements:
What Does Your Voice Say About You?

The five elements: earth, air, fire, water, and metal, are useful to know about and what they say about the tonal quality of your voice.

1. Does your voice draw people to you like a magnet, or does it repel them?
2. Try to be constantly aware of the purpose you're communicating. Who are you speaking to?
3. What is your relationship with these people, this audience? Are you presenting from a stage to a large group and want your audience to do something when you're finished? Or are you healing a relationship with a friend or family member you haven't spoken to in years?

The following are examples of a five-element framework and how you can use it to navigate any form of communication.

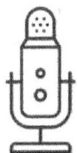

More About Elements of Communication

- *Earth* – Think James Earl Jones and Nina Simone: authority, well-grounded, coming from the gut.
- *Air* – Marilyn Monroe singing "Happy Birthday, Mr. President;" innocent and vulnerable. The air sign is great for balancing if you carry too much fire or metal in your vocal tone.
- *Fire* - Dr. Martin Luther King, Jr., delivered his fiery "I Have a Dream" speech, with passion and dynamic energy.
- *Water* – Preschool teachers and dental hygienists represent the nurturing and compassionate water elements.
- *Metal* – Think Lucille Ball: sharp, clear, able to cut through the din of a crowded room, a nasal voice like a squeaky hinge.

Pro tip: We all use combinations of these tonal sound qualities, frequently leaning toward others. When you can identify your vocal tendencies and the simple act of being aware of any situation, you will have the upper edge by employing these simple tools.

Exercise #10
Seven Chakras to Reduce Stress, Improve Your Health, and So Much More

Finally, the seven energy centers in the body, also referred to as **chakras**. They are known as the base, sacral, solar plexus, heart, throat, third eye and crown chakras. They are the gateways to opening and healing areas that are blocked or in need of healing. Below is a brief description of each chakra, the color it's associated with, how to activate it, and how to use it to uplevel your voice.

1. *Root or base* – physical, identity, grounding, red
2. *Sacral* – sexuality, pleasure, creativity, orange
3. *Solar plexus* – self-esteem, confidence, yellow
4. *Heart center* – devotion, love, compassion, green
5. *Throat* – communication, blue
6. *Third eye* – intuition, imagination, indigo
7. *Crown* – awareness, intelligence, violet or white

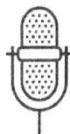

More About Activating Your Chakras

- *Root or base* – Go outside in nature. Take a walk, watch birds, hug a tree—yes, seriously.
- *Sacral* – Listen to anything that calms your nervous system. Being in, around, or listening to water is helpful here.
- *Solar plexus* – Sing songs in the key of E, or simply sing the sound of an open "o" vowel as in the word "Boat."
- *Heart center* – Wear gemstone jewelry, (earrings, rings, necklaces). The soft, pink-colored light of rose quartz encourages gentleness, tenderness, and love. The soft green light of jade brings peace and harmony to the heart.
- *Throat* – Aromatherapy using the tangy fragrance of sage sends healing vibrations into the "seat of language," whereas the refreshing fragrance of eucalyptus oil clears and widens the fifth chakra.
- *Inner eye* – Yantra yoga uses symbols and geometric forms that represent the divine to help you visualize during meditation.
- *Crown* – This center is all about meditation and selfless devotion providing insight into your divine origin to foster a feeling of oneness.

Exercise #11
Recording:
Be the Star You Already Are!!

Welcome to the recording studio! Whether you want to start a podcast, record an EP, (extended play recording) or narrate your book to make it available on Audible, here are just a few tips to get you started.

1. Do your homework. Make sure you've done your pre-production prep before you enter the studio. Work out all the details of your project to avoid wasting anyone's time, which always increases the cost of your project.
2. Practice what you plan to record with a recording device in front of the mirror for family, friends, or a media coach. You'll be glad you did.

When it comes to technology there are so many ways to record any project these days. From as simple as using the microphone and camera on your computer, to fancy equipment, or you can DIY at professional-grade recording studios complete with sound engineers. Choose what works best for you based on your project, resources, and budget.

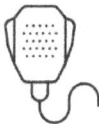

More About Professional Recordings

Potential challenges that could arise prior to recording include everything from going completely blank and forgetting everything you've prepared, to literally removing your voice altogether in an interview situation. Following are considerations to keep in mind.

- Your voice is personal and unique to you. There's a huge amount of fear when it comes to fully showing up and speaking up. Being truly authentic to who you are can be terrifying to share with the world, whatever modality you use.
- The reason these challenges arise is because you're thinking about yourself instead of being of service. "What if I make a mistake?" or, "What will others think?" or, "I don't want to look foolish." When you get out of your own head and get into service, everything falls into place nicely.
- This way of thinking removes the pressure to perform and helps you simply share your purpose from your heart, your passion, and your message that people desire to hear. So, shine like the star you already are.

Exercise #12
Listening:
You Have Two Ears and One Mouth; Use Them in Proportion

Communication is not as easy as it sounds. By now, hopefully you've found several ideas to implement your own way of communicating. This is not just about listening, speaking, or singing. Following are other things to consider when conveying information.

1. **Compassionate communication**. Are you honestly considering input from others, or are you so busy thinking about your response you don't hear anything others have shared?
2. **Body language**. Are you willing to receive information, or are your arms folded across your chest, closing you off from others?
3. **Active listening**. Do you respond to others in a way that validates them in a kind and loving manner versus being judgmental and demeaning?

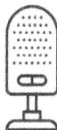

More About Listening and Communication

The human tongue has the power to build up or tear down in an instant. Words can either wound or heal. Here are suggestions to consider when carefully and consciously choosing your style in any given situation.

- Ask questions to help bring all parties involved into alignment instead of barking orders that cause division.
- Speaking in the affirmative leaves a positive effect on the listener, i.e., "Why can't you …" versus "What if we …" or "Please remember," instead of "Don't forget."
- Use "I" statements to show taking re-sponsibility for your own thoughts and feelings instead of "you" statements, which often cause people to become defensive.
- Stay open and neutral giving your full attention, especially when someone is sharing sensitive information. Remember that your feedback is not always neces-sary.
- The less you say can quite often yield a greater return in any conversation.

Exercise #13
Performing/Presenting:
Conquer Fear for Good

If you've gotten this far, and you're still considering getting in front of a room to present your work or jumping on a stage to share your latest project, there are a few things to own to increase your power and presence.

1. Accept yourself as you are. Embrace your unique message and the power within you.
2. Nervousness is normal. Befriend fear and use some of the relaxation and visualization tips shared in this book to diffuse and release anxiety, worry, and perfectionism.
3. Feelings are exactly that. They're not facts; they're often only your perception of a situation. You have the power to convey your feelings using affirmations, meditations, mantras, and other tools mentioned above.

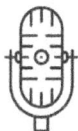

More About Presenting Despite Fear

- Holding onto perfection is poison! Let it go. Get into and stay in service to your audience which automatically takes you out of self.
- Learn how to use space on the stage by coming out from behind the podium, using gestures to emphasize a point, and stimulating engaging audience participation.
- Use the power of the pause (one of the most important techniques used) to emphasize a thought, idea, or call to action.
- Use personal stories to connect with your audience by taking them on a journey of self-discovery or inspiring them to act, join a movement, or make a difference in their own lives.
- Remember to enjoy the ride. None of this is worth it if you're not having fun, so enjoy!

Exercise #14
The Gift of Meditation and Movement

We are spiritual beings having a physical experience on this planet. With so many distractions and multitudes of external forces such as news and social media trying to keep us in a place of fear and lack, it's critical to take care of yourself. If you don't, you can't help others.

1. There are many definitions and forms of meditation. In its simplest form, meditation is the practice of using a technique such as mindfulness or focusing the mind on a particular object, thought, or activity to train attention and awareness to achieve a mentally clear and emotionally calm, stable state.
2. There are as many types of meditation as there are subjects. You can search online for these topics to get started: meditation for stress, sleep, parenting, mindfulness, yoga, breathing, stretching, guided, silent and more.

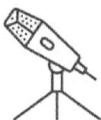

More About Meditation and Movement

Here are some resources to get started if you're new to meditation. Please note that anything you do can become a meditation. I've found that doing dishes and laundry, as much as I don't like spending time on these necessary activities, is actually quite meditative.

- 26 Ways to Access Your Voice Instantly using "I AM" mantra meditations. https://vocalcoachingbysloane.com/26-ways-to-access-your-voice-instantly/
- Deepak Chopra's app for work/life balance
- Mindvalley.com for developing mind, body, and spirit
- Insight Timer app for sleep, anxiety, and stress
- Calm app for guided meditations and soothing sounds like ocean waves or white noise
- www.mindful.org for meditations to replenish cognitive and emotional energy
- Gaia.com for consciousness-expanding videos and courses

Exercise #15
Pick Up the Mic and Get on the Stage!

Congratulations! You made it. Now let's put all this newfound information and energy into practice. Whether you want to sing with confidence at karaoke or connect in a personal and powerful way at home, at work, or with others, here are some accessible ways to do that.

1. For you singers, check out local venues in your area that offer karaoke or open mics, which are usually very encouraging and supportive.
2. If it's speaking/presentation skills you want to practice, visit your local chapter of https://www.toastmasters.org/ where you can also receive feedback. This is great preparation for job interviews and learning how to mentor others.

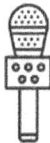

More About Practicing Your New Skills

- Hire a professional vocal coach to guide you. Be sure to ask about the specific method or technique they use. And it's always okay to ask for references from other happy clients they've already served. If they can't provide this simple information, you probably want to continue your search for the right fit.
- Add some fun to your presentation with a skit. Bringing an unexpected element to your presentation is an excellent way to mix things up and engage your audience in a new way.
- Use humor. Comedy and improv clubs are on the rise. Using humor in your presentation humanizes your message. It makes you less threatening, diffuses tension, helps everyone relax and not take things too seriously. Laughter has multiple healing benefits as studies from UCLA are proving with "laugh therapy."

You've finished. Before you go...

Post/Share that you finished this book.

Please star rate this book.

Reviews are solid gold to writers. Please take a few minutes to give us some itty bitty feedback.

ABOUT THE AUTHOR

For more than two decades, Sloane Reali has been helping professionals across industries find confidence through the power of voice. She has helped public speakers, teachers, therapists, doctors, authors, and corporate leaders prepare vocally for their professions.

A leader in her field making guest appearances on television, radio, and podcasts as an expert on the power of voice, clients have used Sloane's services to prepare for television appearances, world tours, and auditions including *American Idol, The Voice,* and *Disney.* Other clients have started their businesses and bands, writing, releasing, and publishing their own books and music, in addition to making guest appearances with music royalty such as David Foster, Lionel Ritchie, and Stevie Wonder, to name a few.

More recently she's gained recognition in the medical community for her work with clients seeking her services after illness or injury has affected their vocal ability, including stroke, cancer, and VCD (vocal cord dysfunction).

Whether working with someone who wants to sing, become a better communicator, or trying to recover their voice after a medical setback, Sloane is a true innovator when it comes to finding your voice, building confidence, and unlocking your potential.

If you enjoyed this Itty Bitty™ book you might also like…

- **Your Amazing Itty Bitty™ Guide to Being TED-Worthy** by John-Alfred Kohler Bates

- **Your Amazing Itty Bitty™ Podcast Book** by Christine Blosdale

- **Your Amazing Itty Bitty™ Fear-Busting Book** by Lucetta Zaytoun

Or any of the many Amazing Itty Bitty™ books available online at www.ittybittypublishing.com

Your Amazing Itty Bitty™ Find Your Voice and Transform Your Life

15 Ways to Instantly Access the Power of Your Voice

Are you suffering from vocal health issues? Are you tired of being passed over for the next promotion or not getting the raise you had planned? Do you feel like you're not being respected in your relationships? If you relate to any of these questions, this book is the starting point for you.

In Sloane Reali's book, she will guide you to discover your voice, feel more confident, and live the life you've always desired. If you're a singer, a public speaker, a partner in a relationship, or a business owner leading a team, this book is aimed at helping you. `

In this book you will learn to:

- Use your breath and inner energy effectively.
- Do proper vocal exercises.
- Use your voice to attract people instead of pushing them away.
- Control the tone of your voice for different situations in your life.

Whether you want to improve your singing, communicate better, or recover from a vocal injury, grab a copy of this must-read Itty Bitty™ book today!